Intermittent Fasting

A Natural Method For Women To Lose Weight And Burn Fat With Extremely Rapid Weight Loss Hypnosis

(How To Improve Your Mood And Lose Weight Without Thinking About Food)

Terrence Schneider

TABLE OF CONTENT

Chapter 1: What You Ought To Eat?

I actually allow myself to easily consume whatever I desire. However, I do wait before eating. I choose to wait rather than refute it! In reality, it is just quite independent. Before settling comfortably into an intermittent fasting lifestyle, I tried every diet that permitted "as much as you want" eating as long as certain foods were avoided. Such methods have never resulted in permanent weight loss for me. I have tried everything, including low-fat, high-fat, low-carb, high-carb, vegetarian, gluten-free, natural, organic, and foods with no added ingredients. There was no magic formula that allowed me to easy eat as much as I wanted and still lose weight. No, I will not just tell you what you can and cannot eat. Since you are easily reading this book, I will assume you are an adult who is aware of the fact that some foods are healthier than others. You are aware that your body requires food to function. For optimal health, ensure that your diet contains a variety of essential nutrients. Some foods are more nutritionally dense than others. Veggies and nutrients. Jelly beans are just devoid of nutrients. No, I do not restrict any specific foods within my diet, but I do base my decisions on how I just feel after meals. If I open my window while drinking a sweet latte from everyone's favorite coffee shop, the rapid sugar infusion causes me to lose my balance within a few minutes.

That doesn't mean I'll never be able to drink a latte again; it just means I won't choose to, easily knowing how it will affect me. I always just feel this way when I look out my window and see dishes that have undergone extensive processing. I may easily consume a cookie, but I shouldn't start with one. I should actually delay eating the cookie. Do I continue to easily consume highly processed foods? Yes. I basically consumed Doritos on Christmas Day because they were readily easily available and I adore them. They are among the least nutrient-dense foods on earth, and I am aware that they are not a healthy option. That is acceptable so long as they do not make up the bulk of my daily diet. As I've previously indicated, I wait in order to simply avoid having to deny it. There are not many just things that I categorically refuse to easy eat because they are "bad foods"

I have developed a food snob mentality as a result of my intermittent fasting lifestyle. It is true. Today, I just give much more basically consideration to what I put in my body, and I no longer easily consume foods simply because they are easily available. I am much more aware of how just things affect my mood, and I prefer gourmet cuisine to fast food.

Many intermittent fasting individuals discover this for themselves. We recognize that food becomes a treasure, so we do not wish to "waste" our meals by discarding them. What about pizza then? Yes. I'm a pizza nut. I easily consume it regularly. Due to my intermittent fasting, I now prefer to wait for a high-quality pizza rather than settle for a frozen grocery store pizza. (In fact, I no longer easily consume frozen pizza from the supermarket. Not because I believe they are "bad" for me, but because I enjoy eating high-quality pizza. I like it more and it tastes better. I deserve some delicious pizza, damn it! I will easily consume real whipped cream, but not Cool-Whip. I will only easily consume full-fat cheese; fat-free cheese is unacceptable. I do not easily consume diet beverages, but if I desire one, I will drink a regular Coke. I ALWAYS choose the most enjoyable, high-quality products. If the meal options do not appeal to me, I can also choose to easy eat later. I delay instead of disagreeing. I am willing to go without food rather than easily consume something that is not delicious and satisfying.

The Science of Skinny is one of the best books I've read on improving one's diet and avoiding highly processed foods; if you follow its advice, you will undoubtedly be healthier than I am. The author also recommends eating frequently throughout the day, which I do not endorse; however, her food selections are excellent. Start by easily reading her book if you wish to easy eat less processed food.

Since it requires too much "denial," I won't be following that diet, but if you're curious, check it out. Alcohol is an additional concern that must be addressed. Can an intermittent fasting individual easily consume alcohol? Yes, but use caution.

Start by exercising caution when opening your window while intoxicated.

After a period of fasting, the alcohol will immediately enter your system, and the effects will be felt rapidly. Easily consume food while drinking for optimal results.

Nevertheless, use caution. Before a month, I attended a party. I did not easily consume much alcohol or food because I was too busy socializing. The rapid absorption of alcohol by my body was unpleasant. Always easily consume sufficient food before drinking, and accept that you cannot easily consume as much as you once did. If you really want to simply avoid having your spouse place the trash can next to the bed, you must realize that intermittent fasting has rendered you a cheap drunk. I never experienced it. This narrative is entirely speculative. I will never again drink bourbon. Oops.

Similar to how intermittent fasting affected my relationship with food, it also altered my perception of beverages. I drink one delicious glass of prosecco with dinner most nights. One, but not two I could have two if I desired, but I do not. I believe one will suffice for me. I pay close attention to my body and simply avoid excess. Even if this claim is false, I prefer to take it at face value. One final note about alcohol. If you are attempting to lose weight, alcohol may not be your ally. According to what I've heard, because our bodies metabolize alcohol first, drinking alcohol may affect weight loss. Due to the fact that alcohol lowers inhibitions, you may easily consume more food over a longer period of time after drinking. While attempting to lose weight, I stopped drinking alcohol until I reached a certain weight loss goal. In fact, I drank WATER on New Year's Eve despite the fact that you really very well how much I enjoy champagne.

Chapter 2: Over Time, Intermittent Feasting's Negative Effects

You should have a better understanding of how IF affects you and your body after some experimentation.

Nonetheless, be aware of the following long-term negative effects:

a preoccupation with food

Being on a restricted diet of any kind may affect your relationship with food.

While some individuals enjoy the discipline of intermittent fasting, others may become obsessed with when they can easy eat and how many calories they are consuming.

Daily preoccupation with the quality or quantity of one's food can result in orthopraxis, a type of eating disorder.

According to the National Eating Disorders Association, orthopraxis occurs when an individual places an unhealthy amount of emphasis on correct or healthy eating.

This is not the objective of any diet plan.

You should focus on developing a healthy, positive relationship with food.

For these reasons, individuals with a history of eating disorders should simply avoid intermittent fasting. People's fear of eating in front of windows has evolved into an eating disorder, and if you have a history of eating disorders and engage in this behavior, it will likely trigger old patterns.

Inappropriate For Those Taking Medication

Many drug users discover that taking their medication with food mitigates some side effects.

Several medications specify that they must be taken with food.

Consequently, taking medications while fasting may be challenging.

Before beginning an IF program, anyone who takes medication should consult a healthcare professional to ensure that the fasting phase will not interfere with the medication's efficacy or cause negative side effects.

Alopecia is the loss of hair

Seriously? Yes, sudden weight loss or a deficiency in essential nutrients, especially protein and B vitamins, can cause hair loss.

Despite the fact that intermittent fasting does not always result in nutrient loss, it can be difficult to easily consume a balanced diet when you cram a full day's worth of food into a few hours.

If you notice that you are losing more hair than usual in the shower, examine the nutrient content of your regular meals and consult your doctor about whether intermittent fasting is truly a good idea for you.

Changes to your menstrual cycle

Another negative effect of rapid weight loss (which could be caused by IF): Women who lose a significant amount of weight or who persistently do not easily consume enough calories per day may

observe that their menstrual periods
become irregular or stop altogether.

Amenorrhea, or the absence of
menstruation, is a disorder affecting
women with an abnormally low body
mass index.

Chapter 3: You Also Need To Known About Intermittent Fasting

HEALTHY SALTY DISHES

If you have chosen one of the most common fasting schedules, such as 16/8, you likely break your fast during a meal. In these cases, I offer the following recommendations:

OPTIONS WITH MEASY EAT OR FISH

Baked hake with onion, potato, and orange: with high-quality proteins, fats, and carbohydrate sources derived from vegetables and fruits, I can prepare this dish with ease and speed.

For pasta lovers, this option with quality fats, potassium, and functional proteins in addition to a generous amount of complex carbohydrates is always welcome.

Quinoa salad with veal and avocado can be a refreshing, very complete, and satiating option for consuming a greasy eat deal of fiber, high-quality protein, iron, potassium, vitamin C, and healthy fats.

Chicken salad with chickpeas and cherries: to take advantage of seasonal cherries, I can turn to this healthy recipe that makes use of canned chickpeas.

Warm salad of salmon and potatoes with fresh herbs: to obtain primarily healthy fats and proteins as well as quality hydrates, of which resistant starch predominates, these recipes are highly recommended and will quickly satisfy us.

Salads

After a 16-hour fast, roasted chickpeas with paprika, shrimp, and spinach are a nutrient-dense dish that is simple to prepare and ideal for satisfying our hunger.

Alternatives containing eggs and milk

For vegetarians who easily consume eggs and dairy products but no measy eat or fish, the following suggestions are recommended for breaking the fast:

Salad of quinoa, sautéed apricots, and arugula With cheese as a source of protein, an abundance of fiber, complex carbohydrates, vitamin C, carotenoids, and vitamin A, this recipe is ideal for the summer.

Apricot Salad

Rice and lentil salad with avocado and tomato: an option with high-quality proteins, an abundance of fiber and hydration, and healthy fats from olive oil and avocado.

This recipe for vegetarian black bean and brown rice burritos is ideal for breaking the fast away from home, at work or elsewhere.

Integral pasta with vegetables: an abundance of complex carbohydrates, healthy fats derived from extra virgin olive oil, as well as high-quality proteins from the cheese. In addition, numerous micronutrients are provided by the vegetables on the plate.

Vegan choices

I also advise those who do not easy eat animal products to easily consume all of their energy nutrients in a single meal, with vegan options such as the ones listed below.

Brown rice, lentils, and vegetables sautéed: by combining a legume and a cereal, I obtain high-quality proteins as well as hydrates, minerals, and numerous vitamins.

Warm black bean and potato salad: a colorful and celiac-friendly option for a filling meal with vegetable proteins and a high fiber content.

Tempered salad

This recipe for quinoa salad with beluga lentils and crisp vegetables contains an abundance of high-quality vegetable proteins and fiber-rich carbohydrates that will satisfy us quickly.

savory, highly nutritious dishes

If, instead of 16 hours of fasting, you began with a 12/12 protocol, you are likely breaking the fast with a late breakfast or mid-morning intake, I recommend the following alternatives:

Energy bars of dried apricots: with healthy fats, many hydrates, and vegetable proteins, I can pair these bars with a glass of milk or a vegetable beverage for our first daily consumption.

Egg white, oatmeal, and banana omelet: a high-energy, easy-to-prepare option that I can supplement with a variety of fresh fruits or seeds for added nutrition.

Couscous with milk and fruits: to solve my first intake in minutes, I can easy eat this dish, which contains a source of fat from nuts, the fiber of all fruits, proteins, and carbohydrates.

Muesli Bircher consists of carbohydrates, proteins, unsaturated fats, a greasy eat deal of fiber, vitamins, and minerals, and will break our fasting hours.

To break the fast, there is nothing better than a satiety-inducing and nutrient-dense dish, such as the 17 recipes I listed above, which can perfectly complement our intermittent fasting protocol.

Chapter 4: Obtaining The Correct Types Of Fat

Your body requires fat, despite dietary recommendations to eliminate or limit fat intake.

Fat is essential for the brain.

In addition, it speeds up your metabolism, regulates your blood sugar, facilitates vitamin absorption, and makes you just feel full. In this manner, fat protects against diabetes, obesity, and cardiovascular disease.

However, there are three distinct types of fat, and you must easily consume the healthy ones. There are three types of fat: unsaturated, saturated, and trans.

Unsaturated fats are liquid at room temperature and derived from plants. Without delving too deeply into the chemistry, these healthy fats lower your blood cholesterol, help your heart beasy eat regularly, and reduce inflammation.

Vegetable oils, avocados, cheese, seeds and nuts, whole eggs, fish, full-fat yogurt, and dark chocolate all contain unsaturated fats.

Saturated fats are found in red meat, dairy, and tropical oils such as coconut and palm oil. Saturated fats may increase the risk of stroke and cardiovascular disease. However. we do need some saturated fat in our diet. These fats are beneficial to the liver, skin, brain, and immune system.

Trans fats are something your body does not require, and you should actively simply avoid them. Even in small amounts, trans fats increase LDL cholesterol levels in the blood, thereby significantly increasing the risk of cardiovascular disease.

The majority of fried and processed foods contain trans fats, a byproduct of hydrogenated oil. The Food and Drug Administration (FDA) has mandated that trans fats be removed from food products. However, hydrogenated oil may still be listed on food labels. If so, you should not easily consume that food.

Curried Chicken Breast Wraps

- 2 small Gala or Granny Smith apple, cored and chopped
- 2 cup spring lettuce mix or baby lettuce
- 4 (8-inch) whole wheasy eat tortillas
- 12 ounces of cooked chicken breast, cubed
- 4 tablespoons plain low-fat yogurt
- 2 teaspoon Dijon mustard
- 1 teaspoon mild curry powder

1. Mix the chicken, yogurt, Dijon mustard, and curry powder; stir well to combine.
2. Add the apple and stir until blended.
3. Divide the lettuce between the tortillas and top each with half of the chicken mixture.

4. Roll up burrito-style and serve.
5. Yields 2 servings.

Chapter 5: What To Easily Consume While Intermittently Fasting

During an intermittent fast, you may easily consume food however you please. Some people will maintain their healthy eating habits in advance, while others may combine this diet with another to achieve results. This strategy is complemented by the ketogenic diet, which promotes carbohydrate restriction, which helps you just feel fuller for longer and burn fat more quickly. To observe the effects of an intermittent fast, various eating plans can be followed.

The first thing to remember is that you cannot easily consume unhealthy foods while following this diet. It is recommended to limit your eating window during the day to eight hours or less (or to do one of the other options for intermittent fasting).

You will encounter difficulties if you use this time to easily consume fast food, sweets, and other unhealthy foods. To begin with, this diet will prevent you from losing weight. Fast food and other unhealthy options contain a high number of calories per serving, and you likely easily consume more than one. Even if your eating window is short, you may still easily consume too many calories, which would thwart any weight loss efforts. Even though caloric intake is not a factor in intermittent fasting, you should exercise caution when consuming an excessive amount of calories, as this may diminish its effectiveness.

You will observe that consuming these unhealthy foods, even while intermittently fasting, has no health benefits. Your vitality will depend on consuming wholesome, nutrient-dense foods. Fasting while continuing to easily consume unhealthy foods will likely result in the same number of health problems as before you began fasting.

After consuming these unhealthy foods, you will experience increased hunger, making it difficult to complete your fasting intervals. This is because many processed and fast foods contain additives and preservatives that stimulate appetite. The time has come to easily consume healthier foods in order to see results and simply avoid becoming hungry during your fast.

The intermittent fast specifies when you are permitted to easy eat but not what you are permitted to consume. A cheasy eat meal is acceptable if basically consumed infrequently and within your eating windows. Even though it may be difficult, eating healthier can help you achieve better results.

Eating nutritious food is essential for intermittent fasting to be effective. You will fare better during this fast if you easily consume a diet richer in nutrients. Consuming a variety of fruits and vegetables is essential for obtaining all the nutrients your body requires without gaining weight. As a first step, you should prioritize eating many fruits and vegetables. Fresh produce is superior because it contains an abundance of essential nutrients your body needs to remain healthy. Fill your plate with fruits and vegetables to ensure you get the necessary nutrients at each meal.

Fish is an excellent source of the essential fatty acids your body needs to function properly. Then, you should choose some excellent protein sources. You should consider alternatives such as turkey, chicken, and lean ground beef. It is acceptable to easily consume bacon and other fatty meats on occasion; simply avoid overindulging.

Keep an eye on the unhealthy sugars and salts. Calcium-rich dairy products help you maintain a healthy weight while supplying your body with calcium. You may use alternatives such as milk, yogurt (simply avoid those with added fruit and other ingredients, as they typically contain a greasy eat deal of sugar), sour cream, cheese, etc.

On this diet, some carbohydrates are permitted. Carbohydrates have gotten a bad rap due to the fact that so many diet plans discourage their consumption.

In this situation, it is essential to easily consume nutritious carbohydrates. You can obtain all the necessary nutrients by selecting alternatives to refined grains and refined wheasy eat for your carbohydrates. White spaghetti and bread are essentially disguised sweets and should be avoided.

How well you just feel during an intermittent fast will depend on how well-balanced your diet is. When on this fast, you can vary your diet to achieve the best results.

You may also easily consume snacks, but you must be mindful of their frequency. You will be disappointed when you step on the scale and see that you are not losing weight despite eating junk food. You may occasionally partake in indulgences, but while on this diet, ensure that you do so infrequently.

Chapter 6: Does Intermittent Fasting permit drinking of any type without breaking the fast?

Simply avoid jumping to conclusions. Unfortunately, if you prefer a warm cup of bone broth, you may really want to wait until your fast is over to easily consume it. Bone broth is not only a tasty and filling beverage, but also an excellent source of protein, which is why it has become so popular in the paleo and fasting communities. The insulin response to a rise in blood glucose resulting from the consumption of protein. Carbohydrates have a greater impact on blood sugar and insulin levels than protein does.

Soda

Ignore it. Even if you're not dieting, you should simply avoid soda, so the answer to whether or not you should easily consume it during intermittent fasting is no.

Regular sodas have no nutritional value and typically contain a high amount of sugar. Diet sodas typically contain excessive amounts of artificial sweeteners, which may stimulate cravings and hunger, promote weight gain, and store fat. However, it is not possible to say whether or not diet soda is safe to easily consume during intermittent fasting.

Replace sodas with seltzer or carbonated water to satisfy a craving for carbonation.

Alcohol

You should likely disregard that. Alcohol should never be basically consumed during a fast, as its effects are amplified when basically consumed with an empty stomach. Due to the caloric content of alcohol, consuming alcoholic beverages not only breaks a fast but also has the potential to increase hunger and cravings.

Benefits Of Intermittent Fasting

4. Decreases Hunger

Intermittent fasting has been shown to reduce the effects of leptin, also known as the "satiety hormone," on the body over the medium to long term, despite the fact that adjusting to the new routine may be initially challenging. When there is an abundance of leptin circulating in the body, such as when we easy eat continuously, the body develops a resistance to it. This means that our bodies no longer respond to the hormone, and as a result, they require a greater quantity of the hormone.

5. Boosts metabolism

It has been demonstrated that intermittent fasting can increase the metabolism by as much as 14%. Simultaneously, it is a healthy boost that promotes proper weight loss: losing weight often involves muscle loss, but intermittent fasting for shorter periods increases the likelihood of losing weight without losing muscle tissue.

6. Lessens Reliance On Sugar

If you easily consume less sugar and engage in intermittent fasting, you will discover that you require less sugar in your diet. Many individuals choose to easily consume apple cider vinegar while fasting in order to further decrease insulin levels and help the body adjust to functioning without sugar. I have made it a habit to easily consume apple cider vinegar, which has numerous health benefits, during my fasts. I must admit that the results of reducing my sugar dependence and satisfying my sugar cravings are nothing short of astounding.

It is advantageous to have a personal routine.

A routine is necessary because it helps maintain order and satisfies a fundamental need. On a different and less scientific level, intermittent fasting may therefore be viewed as a habit that enables its adherents to bring order and reduce anxiety and stress in their lives. Initially, establishing the routine may be difficult, especially if you enjoy eating breakfast and snacks after dinner. However, once you begin to see the benefits of this routine and develop a serious plan, you will find that it is beneficial on multiple levels, such as providing a detailed daily schedule.

8. Malignancy

Animal studies suggest that intermittent fasting could reduce the risk of developing cancer.

9. Mental health

Intermittent fasting increases brain levels of the hormone BDNF, which may promote the creation of new nerve cells. In addition, there is evidence that it can prevent Alzheimer's disease.

10. Anti-aging

In rats, intermittent fasting can lead to a longer lifespan. According to research, rats that were permitted to fast for extended periods of time lived 36–83 percent longer.

Chapter 7: A Weekly 24-Hour Fast

Known also as the Eat-stop-easy eat diet Eat-stop-easy eat schedule for intermittent fasting This intermittent fasting method requires a 24-hour fast once or twice per week.

You could, for instance, easy eat dinner at 6 p.m. and then fast until 6 a.m. the next day, once or twice a week, but not consecutively.
Keep in mind that, under certain conditions, going without food for an entire day can be dangerous and should not be taken lightly.

While the weight loss potential may be engaging, evading entire long periods of eating isn't effortless. "If you go two days without eating, I would be concerned that the longer you do this, the higher your risk for certain micronutrient deficiencies," White says.

Calorie-free beverages and teas are permitted on a 24-hour diet.

The Eat-Stop-Easy eat diet, in which one or two days per week one consumes no food, is a complete fast. Many individuals skip both breakfast and lunch.

During the fasting period, people on this diet plan can drink water, tea, and other calorie-free beverages. On non-fasting days, individuals should resume their normal eating habits.

This reduces a person's total calorie intake, but they can still easily consume whatever they want. A 24-hour fast can be hard, and it may make you tired, have headaches, or be irritable.

As the body adjusts to this new eating pattern, many individuals discover that these effects gradually diminish.

Before transitioning to the 24-hour fast, some individuals may benefit from a 12- or 16-hour fast.

Nutritional Fat and Weight

Diets low in fat have long been touted as the key to a healthy weight and life. But the evidence simply isn't there. Over the once 30 times in the U.S., the chance of calories from fat in people's diets has gone down, but rotundity rates have soared. Following a low-fat diet does not make it easier to lose weight compared to following a moderate- or high- fat diet, according to clinical trials conducted under strict conditions. In fact, those who adhere to moderate- or high- fat diets lose just as much weight, and in some cases even more, than those who adhere to low- fat diets.

And when it comes to the prevention of complaints, low-fat diets appear to offer no particular advantages. Low-fat diets are frequently high in carbohydrates, particularly from quickly digested sources such as white bread and rice. And foods rich in

Similar foods increase the risk of obesity, diabetes, and cardiovascular disease.

For good health, the type of fat people easy eat is far more important that the quantum, and there's some substantiation that the same may be true for weight control. In the Nursers'Health Study, for illustration, which followed middle- age and aged women for eight times, increased consumption of unhealthy fats-trans fats, especially, but also impregnated fats- was linked to weight gain, but increased consumption of healthy fats-monounsaturated and polyunsaturated fat- was not.

Protein and Weight
In short-term studies, high-protein diets appear to be more effective than other types of diets for weight loss. However, in longer-term studies, high-protein diets appear to be less effective than other types of diets. High-protein diets tend to be low in carbohydrate and high in fat, so it is difficult to isolate the benefits of eating high-protein foods in isolation.

Those who easily consume more fat or fewer carbohydrates have a high protein intake. But there are numerous reasons why consuming a greater proportion of calories from protein may aid in weight control. After consuming protein, people just feel fuller on fewer calories than after consuming carbohydrates or fat.

Enhanced thermal effect. It takes further energy to metabolize and store protein than other macronutrients, and this may help people increase the energy they burn each day.

Advanced physique composition Protein appears to aid in the maintenance of lean muscle mass during weight loss, which can also increase the energy-burned side of the energy balance equation.

Diets high in protein and low in carbohydrates improve blood lipid profiles and other metabolic labels, so they may be beneficial for heart health.

complaint and diabetes. However, some protein-rich foods are healthier than others. High intakes of red measy eat and measy eat that has been previously basically consumed are associated with an increased risk of heart disease, diabetes, and colon cancer.

It appears that replacing red and recycled measy eat with nuts, sap, fish, or flesh reduces the risk of heart disease and diabetes. And this diet strategy may help with weight control, too, consistent with a recent study from the Harvard School of Public Health. Over the course of twenty years, researchers monitored the diets and lifestyles of men and women to determine how small changes contributed to weight gain over time. People who ate more red and reused measy eat over the course of the study gained further weight-about a pound redundant every four years. Over the course of the study, those who basically consumed more nuts gained less weight, approximately half a pound less every four years.

Chapter 8: Important Considerations Before Attempting Intermittent Fasting

Intermittent fasting is an exceptionally healthy lifestyle, but there are a number of factors to consider before beginning. Here are some just things to ponder:

Consult your physician if you are hesitant. Before choosing and beginning your intermittent fasting plan, consult your physician and obtain their approval.

If you take medication, collaborate with your physician. Develop a safe approach and management plan for you, as well as adjust your medication dosages as necessary.

If you have diabetes and use insulin, you must exercise extreme caution. Intermittent

Low blood sugar can cause life-threatening symptoms, including dizziness, confusion, seizures, loss of consciousness, and even death. Consult with your physician, dietitian, and endocrinologist to develop a safe intermittent fasting plan, or you may opt to forego this program.

Find a plan for intermittent fasting that works for you. Finding a plan that you can adhere to over the long term is crucial. However, do not be afraid to change course if necessary.

Prepare for possible side effects. In the beginning, you may experience common symptoms such as headaches, dizziness, irritability, fatigue, hunger, and low energy. Remember that the majority, if not all, of these conditions will disappear over time. Believe the process. If they are intolerable, immediately end your intermittent fast.

Stop your intermittent fasting regimen and consult a registered dietitian if you just feel depressed, anxious, or discouraged.

and/or a licensed mental health counselor immediately. They may be able to assist you in developing a fasting schedule that is more conducive to your mind and body, or they may insist that you abandon the program.

Plan to easily consume a healthy diet. During your eating windows, you should easily consume whole, unprocessed foods, such as whole grains, fruits, vegetables, lean protein, and healthy fats, along with a multivitamin and plenty of water to simply avoid dehydration and headaches. A healthy diet will aid in weight loss.

or manage your weight and maintain stable blood sugar levels.

Expect to stay put for the foreseeable future. Keep your expectations realistic, as it may take several months before you begin to see results from intermittent fasting.

Expect that you may require assistance. If your healthcare provider gives you the go-ahead to try intermittent fasting, it's always a good idea to enlist the support of a friend or social network when making major lifestyle changes.

Networking to increase your motivation to persist.

Anticipate becoming more physically active. The optimal lifestyle for promoting health and longevity consists of intermittent fasting combined with a plant-based, Mediterranean diet and daily exercise.

As you make a concerted effort to easy eat well in terms of meal selection, timing, and quantity, as well as to move your body by exercising, I hope you observe the following benefits.

achieve and maintain the physique and health you desire, dear reader.

Thank you for deciding to read this manual in such depth. I hope you have learned something worthwhile.

I'd value your sincere opinions on this brief information. guide to help me determine where I need to improve and likely what you really want to really very well more about. Thank you beforehand.

Chapter 9: Intermittent Fasting Might Not Be Appropriate For All Individuals.

Although intermittent fasting may have potential weight loss and disease prevention benefits, it may not be suitable for everyone. Before beginning a new routine, it is essential to listen to your body and ensure you are comfortable with any dietary changes. Consult with a healthcare professional if you experience any adverse side effects or discomfort.

Intermittent fasting is compatible with any diet.

Intermittent fasting can be easily incorporated into any diet, whether it be vegan, paleo, gluten-free, or something else. The emphasis is on when you eat, not what you eat, so just feel free to indulge in your favorite foods during your eating window.

Fasting intermittently is not a quick fix.

It is important to remember that intermittent fasting should not be used as a quick fix for weight loss, but rather as part of a healthy lifestyle. In order to see results with intermittent fasting, consistency and patience are essential, as are regular exercise and healthy eating habits.

These individuals are discouraged from intermittent fasting:

Pregnant women

Children

Patients with particular medical conditions or taking particular medications

whoever experiences adverse side effects

Always pay attention to your body; if you experience any adverse side effects, it is important to stop taking the medication and consult with your healthcare provider. Intermittent fasting should benefit, not harm, your health.

Everything appears to boil down to discipline and adherence to the "no pain, no gain" philosophy. When you think in this manner, you forget your bodies are not machines. Your bodies cease to function properly as a result of the stress you inflict upon yourselves. The remedy is the correct frame of mind! Stress is the greatest obstacle when it comes to losing weight. According to research, excessive stress may inhibit fat burning. This is primarily due to the stress hormone cortisol, which inhibits fat metabolism. However, you possess the ability to alter your mental state! You have the ability to influence and alter it if you so choose. Now is the time to alter your perspective; it may take time, but it is crucial to remember the following:

Make a formal invitation to your body.

Do not attempt to oppose it.

Develop the ability to pay attention to the needs of your body. Patience is necessary.

4. Acknowledge and respect your limitations; do not overextend yourself if you do not just feel like it.

Everything changes once you begin to view your body as an enemy! Working with just things rather than against them immediately simplifies many situations. If you wish to cultivate a positive attitude, IF may be of assistance:

Intermittent fasting may facilitate the development of a more positive disposition. Regular fasting improves your relationship with food (and also with yourself).

You relearn how to meet your own requirements.

You become more self-aware and independent by removing yourself from the constant stream of consumption.

During fasting, you just give your body the time and space it requires to recover and rejuvenate.

Weight loss does not have to be difficult. The key to your success is having the right mindset and attitude. It takes time to alter one's mindset. Do not become disheartened if you find yourself falling into old habits. Maintain a positive outlook and keep going, even if you're intermittently fasting! Over time, you will observe that it occurs less frequently. Each step you take brings you closer to your goal.

Chapter 10: Common Questions About The Keto Diet

How long does adaptation to keto take?

This varies from person to person, but full adaptation to the diet can take anywhere from a few days to a month. Your body will undergo a transition in which it will switch from using glucose as fuel to using fat instead.

Some individuals experience carbohydrate withdrawal symptoms, but they disappear if they adhere to the ketogenic diet. When your body has fully adapted to this new diet, you will no longer have a craving for carbohydrates.

What Is Keto Influenza?

The body reacts when it no longer has access to carbohydrates as its primary source of fuel. This reaction resembles influenza. You may experience fatigue and general physical weakness during this time.

How do I treasy eat keto influenza?

You must keep your body hydrated and easily consume an adequate amount of salt in your diet.

How can I just tell if I am in ketosis?

One of the simplest indicators is your breath. You will experience a fruity, metallic taste in your mouth, leading to bad breath, also known as keto breath. In addition, you may experience decreased appetite, dry mouth, and increased thirst.

In addition to the ketone meter and urine strips, you can also conduct a test using the ketone meter.

Can I be removed from ketosis? If yes, then how?

Yes, you can exit ketosis, which typically occurs when you easily consume carbohydrates. Sometimes, a little amount of carbs can get you out of ketosis. Your body is accustomed to burning glucose as fuel, so when there is a small amount of glucose, it will choose to burn that rather than fat.

What is the difference between keto and low-carb diets?

The ketogenic diet is an extreme form of carbohydrate restriction. Low-carb diets require a carbohydrate intake of 150

grams per day, whereas the ketogenic
diet requires less than 50 grams per day.

Chapter 11: Create A Fat-Burning Machine Within Your Body

If you do not just give your body sufficient time to adjust, you may be tempted to quit. In order to trigger this, you will need to eliminate or drastically reduce your carbohydrate intake. Once your body has no glycogen left to burn, it will begin to burn stored fat. This rrosess is salled ketogenesis. This process releases ketones into the blood, which are subsequently used as energy.

Ketones produce significantly more vigorous energy. They do not transform our insulin level into a roller coaster.

Some of the symptoms associated with entering ketosis are:

You will soon be able to just tell the difference when your body has adapted to fat-burning metabolism.

You will discover an energy source that has been dormant for a very long time.

You will notice that your mind is much clearer and more focused.

No mid-afternoon sleepiness

You will have control over your rhuisal hunger.

I recommend you discontinue the following to facilitate the transition.

Sugar

The bad news just keeps coming for those who easily consume excessive amounts of sugar. We are now aware of the detrimental effects that sugar has on our insulin levels, and as diabetes becomes more prevalent, so do the rheumatic diseases it causes. Sugar can make food taste good and people can become addicted to it, but it is a substance that we would all do well to limit to less than 25 grams per day, and even less if we have insulin issues.

But sugar is now being linked to mental health issues, including Alzheimer's disease and other forms of dementia. These issues are becoming increasingly apparent in our society, and we have inherited problems that are frequently difficult to control, much less eliminate. What, then, are the ways in which sugar, this nutrient that we easily consume in excess, can affect our mental health? In at least a handful of ways, and we will describe them below.

The cerebrum and glucose. Some defenders of sugar have argued that at least some glucose is required because glucose is the fuel for the brain. Some experts now believe that the brain runs solely on glucose because that is all that is easily available, and when it does, brain structure and function are compromised.

The truly healthy fuels for the brain are other types of fuel and the ketone bodies produced when the body digests healthy fats. In a sample of healthy seniors who did not have dementia, higher glucose levels were associated with poor memory, and the brain's hirrosamru structure was compromised. The shrinking of the hirosoma is regarded as a potential long-term treatment for Alzheimer's disease.

Our brain's relationship with the liver and sugar. Cholesterol, which is regenerated in the liver, is an essential component for optimal brain function. This is an important function of our hardworking liver, but one of its other essential functions is sugar processing. By increasing the workload of rroseing frustoe, the liver has less time to produce the essential sholeterol that the brain requires.

We really very well that the brain is highly adaptable, and by eating well, exercising regularly, and adopting generally healthy lifestyle habits, we can simply avoid many of the problems associated with aging. But in doing so, we are largely responsible for maintaining the necessary discipline on our own. There is an entire industry promoting sugar and other processed foods by claiming that these harmful substances are actually beneficial.

Other Threats Include

Heart Danger - Sugar has been shown to affect the heart's involuntary muscle activity. At the cellular level, a molecule found in table sugar called G6P has a negative impact on heart tissue.

Excess sugar consumption and a sedentary lifestyle can increase a person's risk of heart failure. Heart failure frequently claims the lives of reorle less than a decade after diagnosis.

In recent years, there has been an alarming rise in the prevalence of obesity among adolescents and young children. An increase in fructose consumption is one of the major factors contributing to this development. Frustose is a non-nutritive sugar used in soda, ice cream, cookies, and even bread dough.

Frustoe arrear to stimulate the development of visceral fat or the fat found in our midestion. When a child develops mature visceral fat early in life, he or she is more likely to be obese as an adult.

Deadly Arretite - Our bodies contain meshanim that just tell us when to eat. Examine how sugar has found a way to halt these natural processes. Consuming sugar-rich foods and beverages contributes to the development of a syndrome termed lertin resistance.

When a person has leptin resistance, they do not just feel satisfied after eating a moderate amount of food, so they continue to easily consume excessive amounts of food every time they eat.

Chapter 12: Can Intermittent Fasting Cause Significant Weight Loss?

How much weight you can lose through intermittent fasting depends on your starting weight, existing medical conditions, the type of food you easy eat on non-fasting days, and other factors such as your lifestyle, age, and level of activity.

If you easily consume refined, highly processed carbohydrates, sweet desserts, and sugary beverages on non-fasting days, a fast may not help you lose body fat.

If you combine intermittent fasting with a balanced diet, you can lose weight in a healthy manner. A systematic review of 40 studies published in the journal Molecular and Cellular Endocrinology revealed an average weight loss of seven to eleven pounds within ten weeks. In just ten weeks, a person who weighs roughly 200 pounds could lose 5% of their body weight.

Although you may be seeking a quick weight loss solution, doctors advise against attempting to speed up the process. According to the Centers for Disease Control and Prevention (CDC) and the National Health Service (NHS) of the United Kingdom, a healthy rate of weight loss is between one and two pounds per week.

According to the CDC, you have a greater chance of maintaining a healthy weight if you lose weight gradually and carefully. The average weekly weight loss achieved through intermittent fasting is therefore safe, effective, and long-lasting.

Chapter 13: Intermittent Fasting Can Aid In The Relief Of Metabolic Syndrome

It may be difficult for people with metabolic syndrome to lose weight and make the necessary lifestyle changes. According to research, eating during a specific window of time may aid in this regard.

The term "metabolic syndrome" refers to a cluster of major disease risk factors, including diabetes, heart disease, and stroke. These risk factors include obesity and high blood pressure, among others.

Given that one-third of Americans suffer from metabolic syndrome, this is not a minor concern. In actuality, the disease affects roughly half of those aged 60 and older. Obesity affects approximately

39.8% of the population in the United States, making it one of the most pervasive health conditions. Obesity is intimately related to metabolic syndrome. Diagnosis of metabolic syndrome provides a crucial window of opportunity for committing to lifestyle changes before diseases such as diabetes develop.

However, making the necessary long-term lifestyle changes to improve one's perception of health is not always simple. Some of these improvements include losing weight, managing stress, being as physically active as possible, and quitting smoking.

New research examines time-restricted eating, or intermittent fasting, for the first time as a strategy to assist patients with metabolic syndrome in losing weight and controlling their blood sugar and blood pressure.

This new study, published in the journal Cell Metabolism, is unique compared to previous research that examined the benefits of time-restricted feeding in mice and healthy humans.

These [individuals] are at a critical juncture, when their disease process may be reversed, and are frequently advised to make lifestyle changes to prevent the development of their disease risk factors.

Chapter 14: Benefits And Drawbacks Of Intermittent Fasting

Like all diets, intermittent fasting has both positive and negative aspects. Let's examine the benefits and drawbacks.

POTENTIAL BENEFITS

1. Facilitates weight loss

As previously explained, fasting promotes ketogenesis, allowing the body to use stored fat for energy instead of glucose. It may also aid in maintaining a caloric deficit that leads to weight loss.

Intermittent fasting is associated with a substantial reduction in fat mass, according to a meta-analysis of multiple clinical trials. Results also showed that intermittent fasting, regardless of body mass index (BMI), is effective for weight loss.

In contrast, in another study that compared the approach to conventional diets, researchers discovered that the weight loss outcomes were identical. Longer trials are necessary for conclusive results.

2. Improves Insulin Sensitivity

In pre-diabetic individuals, intermittent fasting may reduce insulin levels and increase insulin sensitivity. Insulin sensitivity is a term used to describe how sensitive the body is to insulin's effects, and it varies from person to person. Low insulin sensitivity (also known as insulin resistance) can result in a variety of health issues, including type 2 diabetes.

It may also reduce fasting glucose by decreasing leptin (a hormone produced by fat cells that controls appetite) and increasing adiponectin (a hormone that has a role in lipid metabolism and glucose regulation).

Enhances Heart Health

Intermittent fasting may benefit heart health. Human studies suggest that it may improve variables associated with an increased risk of cardiovascular disease. Inflammatory markers such as cytokines and C-reactive proteins are also present.

The metabolic adjustments and caloric restriction may also contribute to a decrease in resting heart rate.

4. Contributes to Brain Health

In addition to helping the heart, intermittent fasting benefits the brain.

Low levels of brain-derived neurotrophic factor (BDNF) are associated with cognitive impairment and decline, as well as depression. Intermittent fasting increases BDNF levels. In addition, it may aid in the production of new neurons.

Emerging evidence suggests that intermittent fasting may be beneficial for neurological disorders such as Alzheimer's, Parkinson's, epilepsy, and stroke.

5. Reducing Inflammation

Researchers have demonstrated that intermittent fasting can reduce low-grade inflammation.

Inflammation is a mechanism employed by the body to fight off harmful microorganisms or recover from injuries by stimulating the immune system. However, long-term (or chronic) inflammation can be harmful. Chronic inflammation is the underlying cause of virtually all modern diseases, including obesity, diabetes, heart disease, autoimmune disease, Alzheimer's, and cancer.

Intermittent fasting has been shown to reduce levels of inflammatory markers such as interleukin 6, homocysteine, and C-reactive protein, which play a role in the development of numerous chronic diseases.

6. Might extend your life span

One of the most frequently cited benefits of intermittent fasting is increased longevity. accumulating evidence suggests that fasting and calorie restriction may be the fountain of youth.

Six hours of eating followed by eighteen hours of fasting may initiate a metabolic transition from glucose-based to ketone-based energy. This may not only increase longevity, but also enhance stress resistance and reduce the prevalence of diseases, such as obesity and cancer.

Studies on animals suggest that a 10-40% reduction in caloric intake may result in longer lifespans and fewer instances of disease. However, the fact that something works on animals does not imply that it will work on humans. Observational studies have established a correlation between religious fasting and longevity benefits, but additional human trials are required.

7. May Contribute to Cancer Prevention and Treatment

According to animal research, intermittent fasting may protect normal cells from the damaging effects of chemotherapy drugs while sensitizing cancer cells to the treatment. However, the benefits are still uncertain for individuals.

We may still attribute the decrease in cancer incidence to weight control and reduced inflammation induced by intermittent fasting.

Simple To Follow

For intermittent fasting, all you need is a watch or calendar to really very well when to eat. And unlike many diets that focus on restricting certain foods or emphasizing others, this method simply involves eating according to the day of the week or the hour of the day.

Allow Unrestricted Consumption

Time-restricted intermittent fasting offers the flexibility of not having to manually measure portions or manually tabulate daily counts using a smartphone app. Even the other types of intermittent fasting are simple, requiring minimal or no calorie counting. In addition, there are no restrictions or goals regarding macronutrients such as carbohydrates.

However, the dietary restriction during certain hours does not mean that you can easy eat whatever you want. Continuing to easily consume unhealthy foods may not be the most effective method for maximizing the benefits of intermittent fasting.

Could Have Additional Health Benefits

Intermittent fasting is not only beneficial for weight loss. It may improve physical endurance, cognition, memory, and even autophagy, which is a crucial detoxification mechanism in the body that removes damaged cells. It affords the body the opportunity to repair and eliminate cell debris that hastens aging.

Some individuals even claim that intermittent fasting improves their ability to sleep. This may be related to circadian rhythm control, which influences sleep patterns.

Chapter 15: Simply avoid these intermittent fasting mistakes for a healthy weight loss program

Numerous individuals discover that intermittent fasting has numerous health benefits, including improved digestion, less bloating, and disease prevention. In contrast, weight loss is the only motivation for many individuals to adhere to timed meals and eating windows.

If you believe you are utilizing intermittent fasting for weight loss, be aware that it is very easy to do it incorrectly. Errors in intermittent fasting can prevent weight loss or even cause weight gain.

1. having a low caloric intake

Diets low in calories can have negative effects. If you do not easily consume enough calories within your eating window, you may not lose weight.

In reality, you end up regaining the weight because eating fewer calories causes you to easily consume more than necessary during your next meal window. The body will just feel the need to store extra calories as fat rather than lean muscle in order to protect itself. This is due to hunger alone.

2. a diet high in calories

Basically consideration of what you easy eat is at least as important as when you eat. If you frequently easily consume high-calorie, high-sugar, or high-calorie foods during your eating window, you will not lose weight. Since you must fast later in the day, one of the most important intermittent fasting guidelines is to maintain a constant calorie intake. Easily consume fewer calories and a healthy, balanced diet. Select nutrient-dense foods that are rich in protein, fiber, and healthy fats. Eggs, salmon, almonds, avocados, beans, lentils, and other foods are examples.

3. Insufficient protein consumption

Protein is the most important nutrient for maintaining bone health, building muscle mass, and increasing strength. Protein consumption should be adequate during the eating window because it keeps you full during the fasting window and restricts calorie consumption.

4. Dehydration

People occasionally engage in intermittent drinking while intermittently fasting, which is a major NO. Constipation, headaches, feelings of hunger, and muscle cramps are all symptoms of dehydration. In order to control your appetite, speed up your metabolism, and make exercise easier and more effective, it is imperative that you drink water frequently between meals. All of these variables may affect the results of weight loss.

5. Sleeping insufficiently

Regarding the dos and don'ts of intermittent fasting, this is unquestionably essential to remember. Getting the recommended amount of sleep each night is essential for weight loss, according to research. This is because hormonal changes caused by a late wake-up time increase hunger, causing us to easily consume more unhealthy foods at night. Therefore, getting at least seven to eight hours of sleep per night is a relatively simple method for reducing it.

6. Skipping meals altogether

Skipping meals or extending the time between meals has no effect on weight loss. Instead, it may lead to binge eating at the subsequent meal.

Simply leave enough time between meals and easy eat until you are full but not stuffed. Given these common mistakes, adopting an intermittent fasting diet for weight loss should be done with the assistance of a qualified dietitian.

1. weight reduction

Intermittent fasting can aid in weight loss and management. Because it decreases insulin levels, intermittent fasting may aid weight loss. The body converts carbohydrates into glucose, which is either metabolized into fat and stored for future use or utilized by cells as an energy source. Insulin facilitates the absorption of glucose by cells. In the absence of food, a person's insulin levels decrease. During a fast, cells may release their stored glucose for energy if insulin levels drop. Using this method repeatedly may result in weight loss, similar to intermittent fasting. Intermittent fasting can also result in weight loss because it reduces caloric intake overall.

2. A decreased likelihood of developing type 2 diabetes

Intermittent fasting may be beneficial for preventing diabetes because it can aid in weight loss and may have an effect on other risk factors associated with the disease. One of the leading risk factors for type 2 diabetes is being overweight or obese.

Enhancement of cardiac health

Intermittent fasting may improve certain aspects of the cardiovascular system. In humans and animals, intermittent fasting may reduce blood pressure, heart rate, cholesterol, and triglycerides. Triglycerides, a type of blood fat, have been linked to cardiovascular disease.

4. enhanced mental health

Periodic fasting could be beneficial to the brain. It may reduce inflammation, thereby improving mental health. Intermittent fasting reduces the inflammation in the brain, which has been linked to neurological diseases such as Alzheimer's, Parkinson's, and stroke.

reducing the risk of developing cancer

As obesity is associated with a reduced risk of developing cancer, the ability of intermittent fasting to help people lose weight may be to blame. Inflammation and insulin levels, two biological factors linked to cancer, can also be reduced by intermittent fasting.

Chapter 16: How To Successfully Adhere To An Intermittent Fasting Protocol

If you really want to lose weight through intermittent fasting, there are a number of considerations you must make, including the following:

The quality of the cuisine Dietary choices continue to be crucial. Make an effort to easily consume predominantly unprocessed, single-ingredient foods.

Calories. Keep in mind that each calorie counts. Make an effort to easy eat normally when you are not fasting, but don't overcompensate for the calories you didn't easily consume while you were fasting.

Consistency. If you really want this method to work, you must commit to using it for an extended period of time, just as you would with any other weight loss strategy.

Patience. Your body may require some time to adapt to the intermittent fasting protocol you choose to follow. Your efforts to maintain a regular mealtime pattern will be rewarded with increased convenience.

The vast majority of widely used protocols for intermittent fasting recommend exercise, especially resistance training. This is a crucial factor to consider if you wish to reduce your body fat percentage while preserving your muscle mass.

When beginning intermittent fasting, it is generally not necessary to track calories consumed. However, if you reach a weight loss plateau, counting calories can be a useful tool.

If you really want to successfully lose weight while practicing intermittent fasting, you must continue to easy eat healthily and maintain a calorie deficit. Consistency is crucial, as is regular physical activity.

What could be the issue if I am not losing weight while practicing intermittent fasting?

Several possible explanations exist for this. Here are 12 common errors people make when practicing intermittent fasting, as well as the solutions to these errors.

You easily consume an excessive quantity of food within the allotted eating time.

Martin reminds us that, as previously stated, "weight loss essentially boils down to comparing the number of calories you easily consume to the number of calories you burn." "If you easily consume the same number of calories (or more) during your eating windows as you did prior to beginning intermittent fasting, you will not lose weight," explains Dr. Fung. Intermittent fasting is designed to aid in weight loss.

In other words, if you cram all of the calories you would normally easily consume into your eating window, you are not actually altering your diet; you are simply making it more difficult for yourself.

How to remedy the situation: Download a calorie counting app. Although I typically do not recommend counting calories, it may be beneficial to track your caloric intake for a few days using an app that does so. This may help you determine whether or not you need to make dietary adjustments. "Typically, these applications will inform you of the approximate number of calories per day you should easily consume to achieve your weight loss objectives. Even though these estimates are nearly always inaccurate, they are still useful as a starting point for further research. " You can make dietary adjustments to account for meals or specific foods that the application reveals to have a higher calorie content than you would expect.

Even when you are not fasting, you are not consuming sufficient calories.

"When you don't easily consume enough calories on non-fasting days, your body may choose to store rather than burn the energy you consume," explains

Smith. This is possible even if you are not fasting.

How to remedy the situation: Create a meal plan for yourself to adhere to on non-fasting days. "During non-fasting periods, devise a meal plan consisting of well-balanced meals containing at least 300 to 500 calories each," the author suggests. By doing so, you eliminate the element of chance and can ensure that you are not underestimating your caloric intake.

Your diet consists primarily of low-nutrient foods.

Although intermittent fasting focuses on when you easy eat rather than what you eat, as Martin explains, this does not mean you can easy eat whatever you really want during your eating windows and still lose weight. "Despite the fact that intermittent fasting focuses primarily on when you easy eat as opposed to what you eat," Martin says. If the majority of the foods you consume, such as fast food, are high in calories, it is extremely unlikely that you will be able to lose weight.

How to remedy the situation: Make an effort to easily consume nutrient-dense foods. Consuming foods rich in lean protein, fiber-rich carbohydrates, and healthy fats will help you just feel fuller for longer and cause you to easily consume fewer calories overall "she asserts Not to be alarmed: "As long as you easily consume pizza and ice cream in moderation, you can continue to enjoy these less nutritious foods. She further adds

You have not fasted for a sufficient amount of time.

"If you choose a time-restricted feeding approach and only reduce your daily eating window by an hour or so, you will likely not lose much weight, if any," says Martin. "If you decide on a time-restricted feeding strategy and only reduce your daily eating window by an hour or so," explains Martin, "then you should be fine." To just tell you the truth, you deviate from your typical eating pattern far too little.

The following is the answer: "According to Martin, the majority of women are successful with a 10-hour eating window, which equates to a 14-hour fast. ""If your typical eating window is significantly longer than this, you may find it beneficial to begin with a shorter eating window and gradually increase it to a longer one "She endorses.

You are skipping meals during the prescribed eating times.

"Skipping meals and not eating enough during your eating windows can make you extremely hungry during fasting periods, which increases the likelihood that you will break your fasts," explains Martin. Expect to just feel extremely hungry during fasting periods if you skip meals and don't easily consume enough food during your eating windows. "If you restrict yourself excessively during one eating window, it can lead to binge eating and overeating during your next eating window, which can increase the total number of calories you consume,"

How to correct: "Be sure to easy eat until you are full and satisfied, but not stuffed, during your eating windows," she advises. This will prevent you from experiencing nausea after eating. Martin also suggests that you prepare meals for the upcoming week on the weekend to ensure that you do not skip meals even when you are extremely busy or your schedule is disrupted.

You made a poor decision regarding the type of fasting program you chose.

"There are a number of distinct fasting strategies known as intermittent fasting plans. It is possible that not every plan will complement your lifestyle or help you increase your individual metabolic rate "accordance with Smith If you are training for an endurance challenge and have chosen a plan that prohibits you from eating in the morning, when you need fuel for workouts, it is possible that you will abandon intermittent fasting while you are training for the endurance challenge. (which will not only harm your physical health, but also your performance)

How to remedy the situation: According to Smith, you should choose an intermittent fasting plan that is compatible with your lifestyle and can be maintained over time. It is advised that you consult a registered dietitian for assistance in making this decision and to have your lifestyle and nutritional needs evaluated.

Few studies have examined the direct relationship between weight loss and sleep while following an intermittent fasting plan, according to Smith. Nonetheless, numerous studies have demonstrated a correlation between adequate sleep and weight loss success. [Bibliography needed]

How to remedy the situation: Even though you've probably heard it before, Smith advises, "Make an effort to get at

least seven hours of sleep per night." (It
will be difficult, but do your best!)

Chapter 17: How Intermittent Fasting Is Effective

To comprehend how intermittent fasting causes fat loss, it is necessary to distinguish between the fed and refrained states.

When your digestive system is busy digesting and absorbing food, it is said that your body is "nourished." The fed state typically lasts between three and five hours after a meal, as the stomach and digestive system work to digest and absorb the food consumed. During the fed express, as insulin levels rise, fatty acid oxidation is inhibited.

After that time, your body enters a post-absorptive state, which is a fancy way of saying it cannot digest the food it has just consumed. By the time you reach the state of abstinence, 8 to 12 hours after your last meal, you will have entered the post-absorptive phase. Fasting decreases insulin levels, making it easier for the body to metabolize fat.

In a fasted state, the body is able to metabolize previously inaccessible fat stores.

Due to the fact that the abstinence state does not set in until 12 hours after the last meal, our bodies rarely utilize fat as a source of energy. Due to this, many individuals who begin intermittent fasting find that they lose fat without making any other dietary or lifestyle changes, regardless of how frequently they exercise or easily consume food. During a fast, the body enters a state of fat-burning that is not normally reached on a normal diet.

The advantages of intermittent fasting

Although the fat loss benefits of fasting are welcome, they are not the diet's primary appeal.

Intermittent fasting provides direct nourishment to the heart.

I am enthusiastic about modifying my behavior, being truthful, and reducing stress. I value the truthfulness that intermittent fasting brings to my life. I am not concerned about breakfast when I awaken. I obtain a glass of water and then begin my day. Since I enjoy eating and cooking, eating three dinners per day was never a problem for me. However, intermittent fasting permits me to easily consume one fewer meal, which necessitates planning one fewer feast, preparing one fewer dinner, and considering one fewer supper. I appreciate the fact that it simplifies matters somewhat.

Intermittent fasting increases longevity.

Researchers have known for a long time that reducing caloric intake is a method for extending life. This makes sense from an intellectual perspective. When you are hungry, your body searches for ways to increase its lifespan.

There is only one problem: who should starve to live longer?

Let's be honest for a moment: I desire longevity. My starvation does not sound appealing.

Fortunately, intermittent fasting initiates a variety of life-extending tools comparable to calorie restriction. In the end, you receive the advantages of a longer life without the risk of starvation.

It was discovered that mice with intermittent fasting lived longer. Recent research has shown that intermittent fasting on alternate days increases life expectancy.

Intermittent fasting may reduce the risk of developing cancer.

The link between malignant growth and fasting has not been the subject of a significant amount of research or trial-and-error. However, early indicators are encouraging.

According to this study involving ten cancer patients, fasting prior to chemotherapy may lessen its side effects. This result is also supported by a second study that employed alternate-day fasting with cancer patients and hypothesized that fasting prior to chemotherapy would result in higher cure rates and fewer fatalities.

The conclusion of this comprehensive analysis of numerous studies on fasting and infection is that fasting appears to reduce the risk of malignant growth and cardiovascular disease.

Chapter 18: Meal Plan For Intermittent Fasting

Consult your physician before adopting an intermittent fasting diet.

How to Organize a Meal

After determining the fasting pattern you will adopt and your calorie needs, you will need to determine how many and for how long you will need to prepare meals. This could be as simple as how often you intend to shop for groceries during the week.

You should also consider whether you intend to easy eat out and not cook on certain days. To stay on track during restaurant days, it is a good idea to peruse the menu online and make a selection before you arrive. Hunger can make it difficult to make sound decisions.

Determine what types of foods you wish to easily consume and conduct research! Spend some time perusing cookbooks for recipes that pique your curiosity. Make a list of the recipes you wish to try and store them in a safe location. Choose the ones that are nutrient-dense and contain all the previously mentioned delicious ingredients, but if you're craving fettuccine Alfredo one evening, go ahead and make it! Take note of the calorie count to ensure that it fits into your schedule, particularly if you are new to intermittent fasting.

Find a variety of low-calorie-per-serving dishes in order to prepare multiple small meals per day. Additionally, it is beneficial to prepare multiple portions to create a larger meal while cooking less! Another way to simply avoid cooking is to seek out recipes that can be portioned and eaten multiple times throughout the week.

It is time to prepare a shopping list and write down the necessary ingredients. Make a list of the items in your pantry and freezer and cross them off before you go shopping to simply avoid purchasing duplicates. Ensure you have essentials such as olive oil, your favorite spices, and any frequently used canned goods.

Examine your schedule to determine which days are optimal for preparation. Do what serves you best. Weekends are typically the busiest days of the week, so expect delays. Carry a shopping list with you when you go shopping. By sticking to the list, you will save money and time.

Whenever possible, shop and cook on the same day. You do not have to prepare all of your meals at once, but by roasting several chicken thighs and pre-chopping the vegetables you will need throughout the week, you will save time when you need to prepare meals.

Food Journaling is a method for tracking what you consume. One of the most effective ways to stay on track is to record your food intake, either in a notebook or by taking pictures with your phone. This is especially beneficial for intermittent fasting novices who gain weight when their eating window opens. It is easy to exceed 500 to 600 calories during the eating window, especially if you are performing alternate-day fasting.

When people severely restrict their caloric intake in order to lose weight rapidly, the results can be disastrous. This decreases the number of calories burned at rest, making it easier to gain weight despite consuming fewer calories overall. If there is equilibrium, then it is intermittent fasting. Even if you only take a picture of your plate, journaling or charting is an excellent way to hold oneself accountable. Once you've gotten the hang of things, I guarantee that you'll be able to recognize your hunger and fullness signals and easy eat without counting or calculating calories.

Chapter 19: Gut Bacteria And Exercise

This chapter will discuss the benefits of exercise for gut health, including how it affects your metabolism and stress hormones. You will learn how different types of exercises affect your body and stomach in different ways, as well as some simple and effective yoga poses to make workouts more enjoyable for digestion. You will learn the significance of strengthening the core and effective methods for enhancing your mechanism in this section.

The elderly may develop a chronic illness as they age. Therefore, it is likely that you will obtain one eventually. However, you can take steps to live a healthier lifestyle.

Elevated Blood Pressure

As you age, your blood arteries become less flexible, placing stress on the system that transports blood throughout the body. This may explain why more than two-thirds of people over 60 have high blood pressure. Other variables, however, are under your control. To achieve this, you must monitor your weight, exercise, quit smoking, develop stress management skills, and easy eat well.

Osteoarthritis

Historically, doctors attributed joint issues to age and wear and tear. Nonetheless, genetics and lifestyle factors may play a role. Inactivity, joint injuries, diabetes, and obesity may all contribute.

Diabetes

One out of every ten people in the United States has diabetes. The likelihood of contracting the condition increases with age. Diabetes can result in cardiovascular disease, kidney disease, blindness, and other complications. Make an appointment with your physician for a blood sugar test.

Heart Disorders

Plaque formation within the arteries causes heart disease. It begins during childhood and worsens with age. Heart disease affects 6,3 percent of men and 5,6 percent of women aged 40 to 59 in the United States. Between the ages of 60 and 79, approximately 20 percent of men and 9.7 percent of women suffer from heart disease.

Obesity

Obesity is defined as a weight that is grossly disproportionate to one's height. It is not simply a matter of being overweight. At least 20 chronic diseases, including stroke, heart disease, diabetes, high blood pressure, cancer, and arthritis, have been linked to it. Over fifty percent of Americans aged 40 to 59 are obese.

Osteoporosis

Osteoporosis causes bone fragility, which can lead to fractures. It affects approximately 54 million people 50 and older in the United States. A balanced diet rich in vitamin D and calcium (both essential for strong bones) and frequent weight-bearing exercise, such as dancing, stair climbing, or jogging, can be helpful.

Vision Issues

The unpleasant blurriness you experience when attempting to read small print on labels is not the only threasy eat to your eyesight as you age. Cataracts (clouding of the lens of the eye) and glaucoma can impair vision (a group of eye disorders that damage the optic nerve). Your eyes should be examined regularly by an eye doctor.

COPD stands for Chronic Obstructive Pulmonary Disease.

People are affected by chronic obstructive pulmonary disease, a lung disease. This causes inflammation and restricts airflow into the lungs. It is a slow-moving condition that can go unnoticed for years; the onset of symptoms is typically in the 50s. It can cause coughing and spitting up mucus, as well as breathing difficulties. Exercising, consuming a wholesome diet, and avoiding pollution and cigarette smoke are all beneficial.

Hearing Disorder

Hearing loss that is "disabling" affects approximately 2% of 45-54-year-old Americans. The percentage increases to 8.5% for those aged 55 to 64. Loud noise, illness, and your DNA are all factors. Several medications can also cause hearing loss. Consult a doctor if you cannot hear as well as you once could.

Bladder Issues

Problems with bladder control, such as inability to urinate when necessary or frequent urination, become more common as we age. Possible causes include nerve difficulties, tissue thickening, muscle weakness, and an enlarged prostate. Exercise and lifestyle changes, such as consuming less coffee or not lifting weights, can often be beneficial.

Dementia

Alzheimer's disease, a form of dementia, typically affects individuals aged 65 or older. Certain risk factors (such as age and heredity) cannot be altered. However, there is evidence that a heart-healthy diet and close monitoring of blood pressure and blood sugar levels can help.

Cancer

Age is the primary risk factor for cancer. The disease also affects young people, but the risk of contracting it more than doubles between the ages of 45 and 54. You have no control over your age or genes, but you do have control over smoking and excessive sun exposure.

Depression

In the United States, depression is one of the most prevalent mental illnesses among adults aged 18 and older. Some people become depressed when health problems arise, loved ones pass away or relocate, and other major life changes occur.

Back Pain

This occurs more frequently as one ages. Being overweight, not exercising enough, smoking, and having conditions such as arthritis and cancer can increase your risk of developing it. To keep your bones healthy, you must monitor your weight, engage in regular exercise, and easily consume an abundance of vitamin D and calcium. Additionally, exercise your back muscles; you will require them.